MW01227034

Healthy Keto Diet Cookbook

Easy Keto Diet Recipes for Keep Healthand Lose Weight

Laura J. Amin

Sommario

Introduction

Are you trying to find a simple means to cook healthy meals in the convenience of your very own home? Are you looking for simple kitchen devices that will aid you prepare some rich and also scrumptious dishes for you and your liked ones? Well, if that's the case, then this is the best guide you might utilize.This food preparation guide offers to you the most effective as well as most cutting-edge cooking device offered these days. We're speaking about the immediate pot This original and also valuable pot has gotten so many followers throughout the world due to the fact that it's so easy to use and also due to the fact that it can assist you prepare so many scrumptious meals. You can prepare very easy breakfasts, lunch dishes, treats, appetizers, side dishes, fish as well as seafood, meat, fowl, veggie and treat dishes immediate pot.This brings us to the second part of this overview. This journal concentrates on utilizing the immediate pot to make the most effective Ketogenic recipes. The Ketogenic diet regimen is far more than a straightforward weight management program. It's a lifestyle that will improve your health and wellness as well as the means you look.

This low-carb as well as high-fat diet regimen will certainly obtain your body to a state of ketosis. The diet assistance you generate even more ketones as well as a result it will certainly improve your metabolic process as well as your power degrees.The Ketogenic diet will certainly show its multiple advantages in a matter of mins as well as it will certainly aid you look better.

Ketogenic Instant Pot Snack and Appetizer Recipes

Cod and Tomatoes

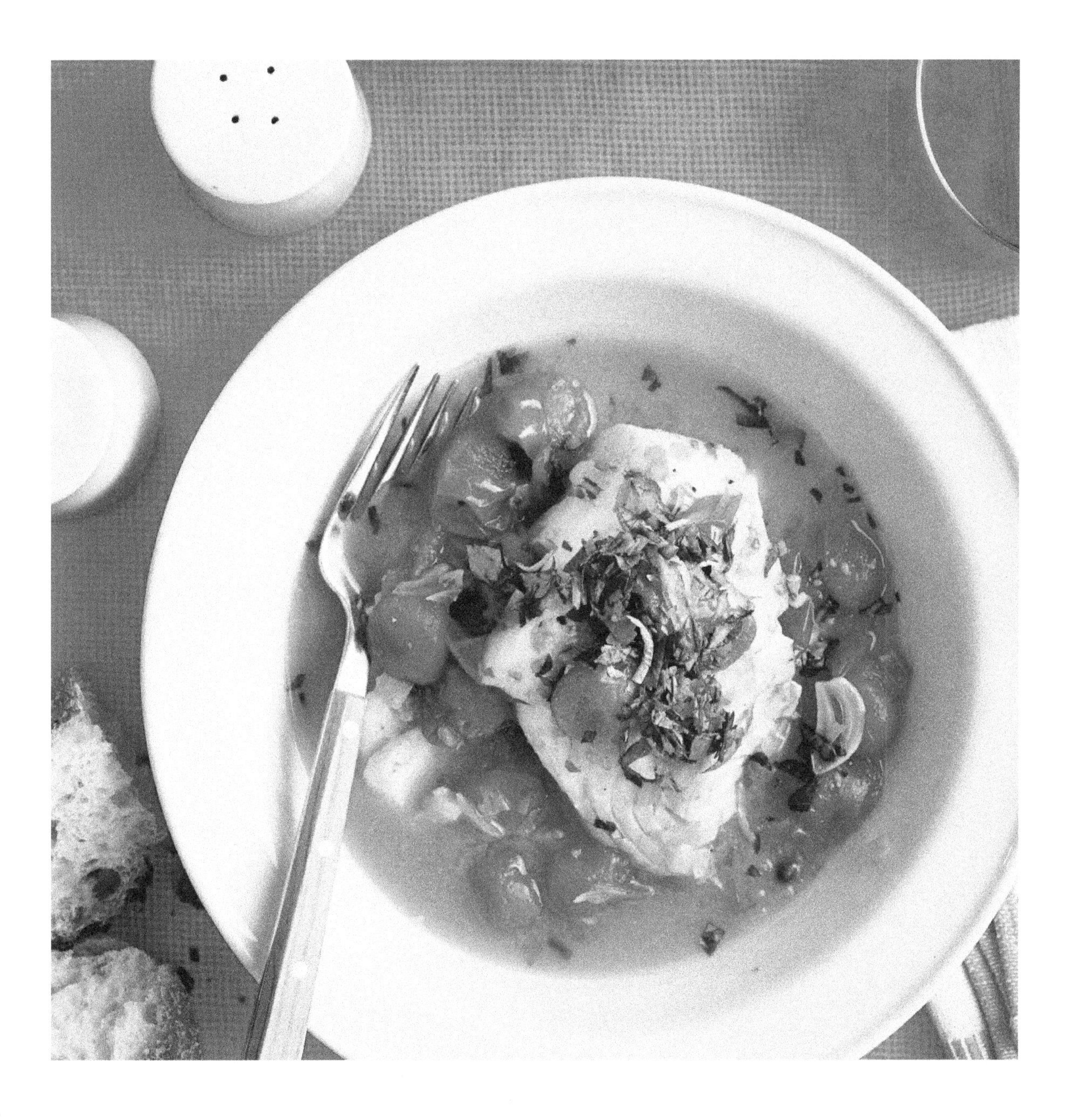

Preparation time: 10 minutes

Cooking time: 15 minutes

Servings: 4

Ingredients:

- 4 cod fillets, boneless and skinless
- ¼ cup chicken stock
- 2 tablespoons olive oil
- Juice of 1 lemon
- 2 shallots, chopped
- 3 tomatoes, cubed
- 4 thyme springs, chopped
- A pinch of salt and black pepper

Directions:

Set the instant pot on Sauté mode, add the oil, heat it up, add the shallots and cook for 2 minutes.Add the rest of the ingredients, put the lid on and cook on High for 12 minutes. Release the pressure naturally for 10 minutes, divide everything between plates and serve.

Nutrition: calories 232, fat 16.5, fiber 1.1, carbs 4.8, protein 16.5

Fish Saag

Preparation time: 10 minutes

Cooking time: 5 minutes

Servings: 4

Ingredients:

- 1 teaspoon tomato paste
- ½ white onion, diced
- 4 tablespoons coconut milk
- ½ teaspoon ginger, minced
- ¼ teaspoon garlic powder
- ½ teaspoon garam masala
- ½ teaspoon ground turmeric
- 1 cup spinach, chopped

- ¼ teaspoon salt
- ½ cup of water
- 12 oz haddock fillet
- 1 teaspoon olive oil
- ¼ teaspoon ground black pepper

Directions:

Put in the blender: tomato paste, diced onion, ginger, garlic powder, garam masala, ground turmeric, and chopped spinach. Blend the mixture until is smooth (appx.2 minutes). Then add water and pulse it for 10 seconds. Pour the liquid in the instant pot. Insert the steamer rack over it. Brush the haddock fillet with olive oil and sprinkle with salt and ground black pepper. Place the fish on the foil. Fold the foil to get the fish package and transfer it on the steamer rack. Close and seal the lid. Cook the fish saag for 5 minutes on steam mode (high pressure). When the time is over, make a quick pressure release and remove the fish. Cut the haddock fillet into the servings and place it on the plate. Top every fish serving with spinach sauce (from the instant pot).

Nutrition: calories 151, fat 5.6, fiber 1, carbs 3.2, protein 21.5

Cod and Cilantro Sauce

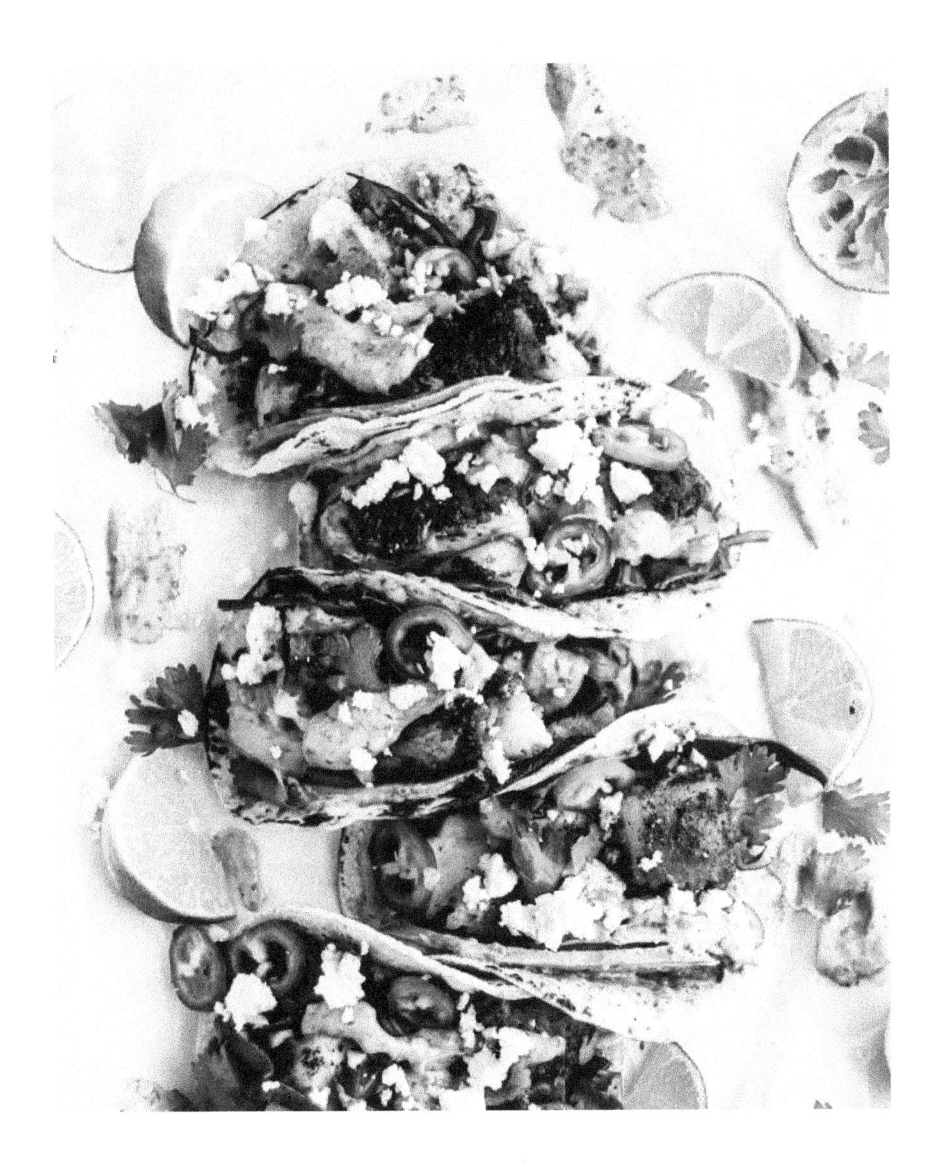

Preparation time: 5 minutes

Cooking time: 15 minutes

Servings: 4

Ingredients:

- 4 cod fillets, boneless
- ¼ cup chicken stock
- 1 tablespoon ghee, melted
- 1 tablespoon ginger, grated
- Salt and black pepper to the taste
- Juice of 1lemon
- 2 tablespoons cilantro, chopped

Directions:

In a blender, combine the ghee with the ginger, lemon juice and cilantro and blend well. In your instant pot, combine the cod with the cilantro sauce, salt, pepper and the stock, put the lid on and cook on High for 15 minutes. Release the pressure fast for 5 minutes, divide everything between plates and serve.

Nutrition: calories 188, fat 12.8, fiber 0.2, carbs 2.2, protein 16.8

Brazilian Fish Stew

Preparation time: 10 minutes

Cooking time: 14 minutes

Servings: 6

Ingredients:

- 6 halibut fillet, chopped (6 oz each fish fillet)
- 1 tablespoon almond butter
- 1 tablespoon lemon juice
- 1 teaspoon fresh parsley, chopped
- 1 white onion, diced
- 1 green bell pepper, chopped
- 2 garlic cloves, diced
- 1 teaspoon tomato paste

- 1 cup chicken broth
- 3 tablespoons coconut milk
- 1 teaspoon ground coriander
- 1 teaspoon paprika
- ½ teaspoon white pepper
- ¼ teaspoon chili powder

Directions:

Make the stew sauce: combine together almond butter, lemon juice, parsley, onion, bell pepper, diced garlic, tomato paste, chicken broth, coconut milk, ground coriander, paprika, white pepper, and chili powder. Then transfer the mixture in the instant pot and close the lid. Cook the ingredients for 8 minutes on manual mode (high pressure). Then allow the natural pressure release and open the lid. Stir the stew sauce well and set sauté mode for 6 minutes. Cook the stew on sauté mode for 1 minute and then add chopped halibut fillets. Close the lid and sauté the stew for the remaining 5 minutes.

Nutrition: calories 247, fat 7.7, fiber 1.2, carbs 4.8, protein 38.1

Salmon and Black Olives Mix

Preparation time: 5 minutes

Cooking time: 15 minutes

Servings: 4

Ingredients:

- 1 pound salmon fillets, boneless, skinless and cubed
- 1 cup black olives, pitted and chopped
- 1 cup kalamata olives, pitted and chopped
- 2 garlic cloves, minced
- 1 tablespoon olive oil
- A pinch of salt and black pepper
- ¼ cup chicken stock
- 1 tablespoon parsley, chopped

Directions:

Set the instant pot on Sauté mode, add the oil, heat it up, add the fish and sear for 2 minutes on each side. Add the rest of the ingredients, put the lid on and cook on High for 10 minutes. Release the pressure fast for 5 minutes, divide everything between plates and serve.

Nutrition: calories 261, fat 17.6, fiber 2.2, carbs 4.8, protein 22.5

Fish Casserole

Preparation time: 5 minutes

Cooking time: 15 minutes

Servings: 6

Ingredients:

- 1 cup white mushrooms, chopped
- 1 tablespoon coconut oil
- 1 teaspoon ground black pepper
- 1 tablespoon fresh cilantro, chopped
- 1 cup whipped cream
- 1-pound cod, chopped
- 2 oz Parmesan, grated
- 1 teaspoon dried oregano

Directions:

Toss coconut oil in the instant pot and melt it on sauté mode. Then add chopped white mushrooms and cook for 5 minutes. Stir them from time to time. After this, add ground black pepper, dried oregano, and chopped cod. Stir the ingredients with the help of the spatula and cook for 2 minutes. Then add fresh cilantro and whipped cream. Mix up the casserole and cook it for 3 minutes. Then top the meal with Parmesan and close the lid.

Cook the casserole for 5 minutes.

Nutrition: calories 192, fat 11.2, fiber 0.3, carbs 1.7, protein 21.2

Coriander Cod Mix

Preparation time: 5 minutes

Cooking time: 15 minutes

Servings: 4

Ingredients:

- 4 cod fillets, boneless and skinless
- 1 cup coconut cream
- 2 spring onions, sliced
- 2 garlic cloves, minced
- 1 tablespoons coriander, chopped
- A pinch of salt and black pepper
- 2 tablespoons lime juice

Directions:

In your instant pot, combine the trout with the cream and the rest of the ingredients, put the lid on and cook on High for 15 minutes. Release the pressure fast for 5 minutes, divide everything between plates and serve.

Nutrition: calories 297, fat 24.3, fiber 1.6, carbs 5.4, protein 17.6

Salmon Pie

Preparation time: 15 minutes

Cooking time: 20 minutes

Servings: 4

Ingredients:

- 10 oz salmon fillet, chopped
- ½ teaspoon ground coriander
- ½ teaspoon salt
- ½ cup green peas
- ½ cup heavy cream
- 1 teaspoon coconut oil
- 1 teaspoon sesame oil
- ½ cup almond meal

- 2 tablespoons butter, softened
- 1 cup water, for cooking

Directions:

Toss the coconut oil in the instant pot bowl and melt it on sauté mode. When the oil is melted, add chopped salmon fillet. Sprinkle it with coriander and cook for 1 minute from each side. After this, add salt, green peas, and heavy cream. Close the lid and sauté the fish for 3 minutes. Meanwhile, make the pie dough: mix up together almond meal and butter. Knead the dough. Brush the instant pot baking pan with sesame oil. Then place the dough inside and flatten it in the shape of the pie crust. Put the salmon fillet mixture (stuffing) inside the pie crust and flatten it. Cover the pie with foil and secure the edges. Then clean the instant pot and pour water inside. Arrange the steamer rack and put the pie on it. Cook the salmon pie for 15 minutes on Manual mode (high pressure). When the time is over, make a quick pressure release and open the lid. Remove the foil and let the pie cool for 10-15 minutes. Cut it into the servings. Transfer the serving in the table with the help of the spatula.

Nutrition: calories 300, fat 24, fiber 2.4, carbs 5.6, protein 17.6

Cod and Zucchinis

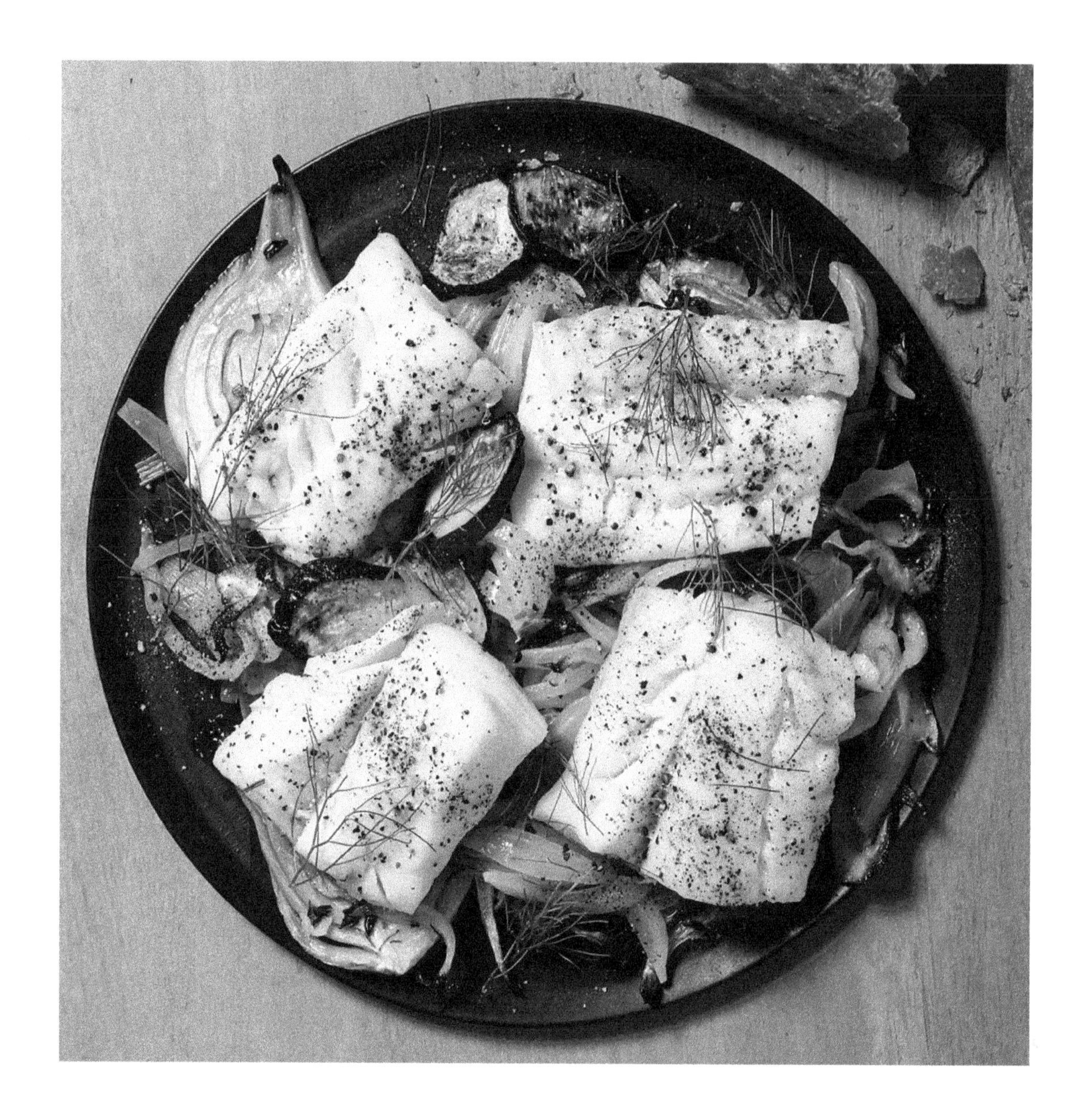

Preparation time: 5 minutes

Cooking time: 15 minutes

Servings: 4

Ingredients:

- 4 cod fillets, boneless and skinless
- 2 zucchinis, sliced
- 1 tablespoon avocado oil
- 2 garlic cloves, minced
- 1 tablespoon sweet paprika
- Salt and black pepper to the taste
- 1 tablespoon parsley, chopped
- ½ cup veggie stock

Directions:

Set the instant pot on Sauté mode, add the oil, heat it up, add the garlic and sauté for 2 minutes. Add the rest of the ingredients, put the lid on and cook on High for 12 minutes. Release the pressure naturally for 5 minutes, divide the mix between plates and serve.

Nutrition: calories 182, fat 10.4, fiber 1.9, carbs 6.2, protein 17.5

Pesto Salmon

Preparation time: 10 minutes

Cooking time: 10 minutes

Servings: 3

Ingredients:

- 9 oz salmon fillet (3 oz every salmon fillet)
- 3 teaspoons pesto sauce
- 1 teaspoon butter
- 2 tablespoons organic almond milk

Directions:

Melt butter in sauté mode. Meanwhile, mix up together almond milk and pesto sauce. Brush the salmon fillets with pesto mixture from both sides and put in the melted butter. Cook the fish for 3 minutes from each side on sauté mode.

Nutrition: calories 166, fat 9.9, fiber 0.1, carbs 3, protein 17.3

Paprika Trout

Preparation time: 5 minutes

Cooking time: 12 minutes

Servings: 4

Ingredients:

- 4 trout fillets, boneless and skinless
- ½ cup chicken stock
- A pinch of salt and black pepper
- ½ teaspoon oregano, dried
- 2 teaspoons sweet paprika
- 1 tablespoon chives, chopped

Directions:

In your instant pot, combine the trout with the rest of the ingredients, put the lid on and cook on High for 12 minutes. Release the pressure fast for 5 minutes, divide the mix between plates and serve.

Nutrition: calories 132, fat 5.5, fiber 0.5, carbs 0.9, protein 16.8

Tuna Salad

Preparation time: 15 minutes

Cooking time: 5 minutes

Servings: 5

Ingredients:

- 3 eggs
- ½ red onion, diced
- ½ teaspoon minced garlic
- 1 avocado, pitted, peeled, chopped
- 1 celery stalk, chopped
- 3 tablespoons ricotta cheese
- 1 teaspoon lemon juice
- ½ teaspoon ground paprika

- 8 oz tuna, canned
- 1 cup water, for cooking

Directions:

Pour water and insert the steamer rack in the instant pot. Put eggs on the rack and close the lid. Cook the eggs on steam mode for 5 minutes. Allow the natural pressure release for 5 minutes. The cool the eggs in cold water. Peel the eggs. Meanwhile, make the salad sauce: mix up together ricotta cheese, lemon juice, minced garlic, and ground paprika. In the salad bowl combine together, onion, avocado, and celery stalk. Shred the canned tuna and add it in the salad bowl too. After this, add salad sauce. Chop the eggs and add in the salad too. Mix up the cooked meal.

Nutrition: calories 223, fat 14.9, fiber 3.1, carbs 5.5, protein 17.4

Lime Shrimp

Preparation time: 5minutes

Cooking time: 8 minutes

Servings: 4

Ingredients:

- 1 pound shrimp, peeled and deveined
- Zest of 1 lime, grated
- Juice of 1 lime
- 1 cup chicken stock
- ¼ cup cilantro, chopped
- A pinch of salt and black pepper

Directions:

In your instant pot, combine the shrimp with the rest of the ingredients, put the lid on and cook on High for 8 minutes. Release the pressure fast for 5 minutes, divide the shrimp between plates and serve with a side salad.

Nutrition: calories 138, fat 3.8, fiber 0, carbs 2, protein 26

Tandoori Salmon

Preparation time: 15 minutes

Cooking time: 3 minutes

Servings: 2

Ingredients:

- ½ teaspoon garam masala
- ½ teaspoon ground paprika
- 1 teaspoon minced ginger
- ½ teaspoon ground turmeric
- ½ teaspoon salt
- ½ teaspoon chili powder
- ½ teaspoon minced garlic
- 1 tablespoon lemon juice

- 1 tablespoon olive oil
- 10 oz salmon fillet
- 1 cup water, for cooking

Directions:

Cut the salmon fillet into 2 servings. After this, in the mixing bowl combine together garam masala, paprika, minced ginger, ground turmeric, salt, chili powder, minced garlic, lemon juice, and olive oil. Stir the mixture until smooth. Rub the salmon fillets with the spice mixture and arrange it in the steamer rack. Pour water in the instant pot and insert the steamer rack with salmon inside. Close the lid and cook the meal for 3 minutes on steam mode (high pressure). When the time is over, make a quick pressure release and open the lid.

Nutrition: calories 259, fat 16.1, fiber 0.7, carbs 2.1, protein 27.9

Trout and Radishes

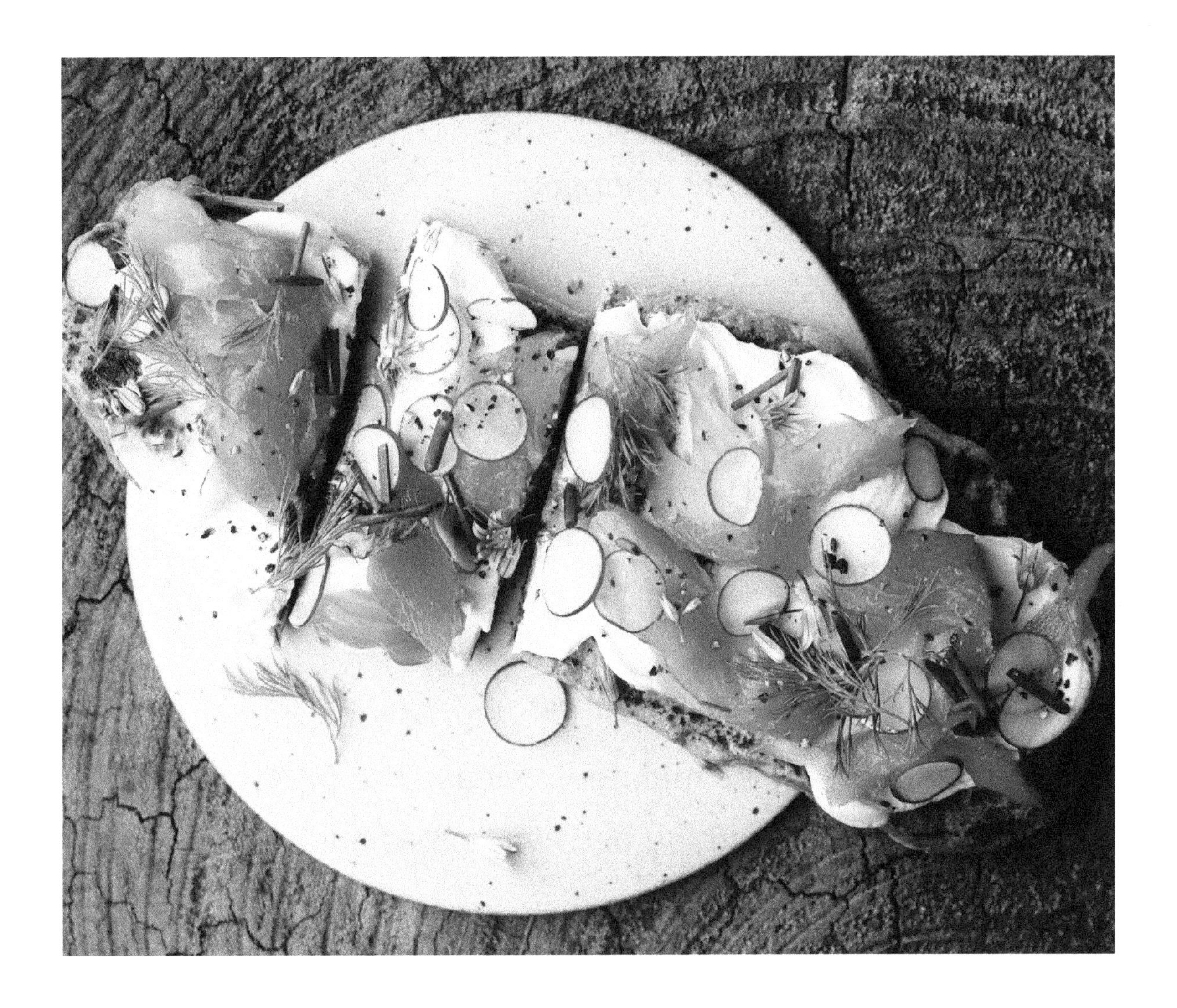

Preparation time: 5 minutes

Cooking time: 12 minutes

Servings: 4

Ingredients:

- 4 trout fillets, boneless and skinless
- A pinch of salt and black pepper
- 1 tablespoon parsley, chopped
- 2 tablespoons tomato passata
- 2 cups red radishes, sliced

Directions:

In your instant pot, combine all the ingredients, put the lid on and cook on High for 12 minutes. Release the pressure fast for 5 minutes, divide everything between plates and serve.

Nutrition: calories 129, fat 5.3, fiber 1.1, carbs 2.5, protein 17

Cheese Melt

Preparation time: 10 minutes

Cooking time: 6 minutes

Servings: 2

Ingredients:

- 2 low carb tortillas
- ¼ cup Cheddar cheese, shredded
- 4 oz tuna, canned
- 1 teaspoon cream cheese
- ½ teaspoon Italian seasonings
- 1 teaspoon sesame oil

Directions:

Shred the tuna and mix it with Italian seasonings and cream cheese. Then spread the mixture over the tortillas. Top the mixture with Cheddar cheese and fold into the shape of pockets. Pour sesame oil in the instant pot and heat it up on sauté mode for 2 minutes. Then arrange the cheese pockets in the instant pot and cook them for 2 minutes from each side. Transfer the cooked meal in the serving plates. It is recommended to eat the cheese melts immediately after cooking.

Nutrition: calories 272, fat 14.5, fiber 7, carbs 12.4, protein 21.7

Cod and Broccoli

Preparation time: 5 minutes

Cooking time: 15 minutes

Servings: 4

Ingredients:

- 4 cod fillets, boneless and skinless
- A pinch of salt and black pepper
- 1 pound broccoli florets
- 2 tablespoon tomato passata
- 1 cup chicken stock
- 1 tablespoon cilantro, chopped

Directions:

In your instant pot, combine all the ingredients, put the lid on and cook on High for 15 minutes. Release the pressure fast for 5 minutes, divide the mix between plates and serve.

Nutrition: calories 197, fat 10, fiber 3.1, carbs 4.3, protein 19.4

Prosciutto Shrimp Skewers

Preparation time: 15 minutes

Cooking time: 4 minutes

Servings: 7

Ingredients:

- 1-pound shrimps, peeled
- 4 oz prosciutto, sliced
- ½ teaspoon olive oil
- ¼ teaspoon chili powder
- 1 cup water, for cooking

Directions:

Wrap every shrimp in prosciutto and string on the skewers. Then sprinkle the shrimps with olive oil and chili powder. Pour water in the instant pot and arrange the steamer rack. Place the shrimp skewers in the steamer and close the lid. Cook the meal for 4 minutes on manual mode (high pressure). When the time is over, make a quick pressure release and open the lid. Transfer the cooked shrimp skewers on the plate.

Nutrition: calories 104, fat 2.4, fiber 0, carbs 1.3, protein 18.2

Rosemary Trout and Cauliflower

Preparation time: 10 minutes

Cooking time: 15 minutes

Servings: 4

Ingredients:

- 4 trout fillets, boneless and skinless
- ½ cup veggie stock
- 2 garlic cloves, minced
- 2 cups cauliflower florets
- 1 tablespoon avocado oil
- A pinch of salt and black pepper
- 1 tablespoon rosemary, chopped

Directions:

Set the instant pot on Sauté mode, add the oil, heat it up, add the garlic and sauté for 2 minutes. Add the rest of the ingredients, put the lid on and cook on High for 13 minutes. Release the pressure naturally for 10 minutes, divide the mix between plates and serve.

Nutrition: calories 140, fat 5.9, fiber 1.8, carbs 3.9, protein 17.7

Lime Salmon Burger

Preparation time: 10 minutes

Cooking time: 8 minutes

Servings: 6

Ingredients:

- 14 oz salmon fillet
- 1 teaspoon mustard
- ½ teaspoon lime zest, grated
- 1 tablespoon lime juice
- ½ teaspoon chives, chopped
- ½ teaspoon ground black pepper
- ½ teaspoon cayenne pepper
- 1 teaspoon olive oil

- ¼ teaspoon ground coriander
- 12 Cheddar cheese slices

Directions:

Chop the salmon fillet and put it in the blender. Blend the fish until smooth and transfer it in the mixing bowl. Add mustard, lime zest, lime juice, chives, ground black pepper, cayenne pepper, and ground coriander. Stir the mixture with the help of the spoon and make 6 burgers, Brush the instant pot with olive oil. Place the salmon burgers in the instant pot in one layer. Set sauté mode and cook them for 5 minutes. Then flip the burgers on another side and cook for 3 minutes more. When the fish burgers are cooked, transfer them on the plate and cool for 5 minutes. Then place every salmon burger on the cheese slice and top with the remaining cheese slice. Pierce every burger with a toothpick.

Nutrition: calories 324, fat 23.6, fiber 0.2, carbs 1.2, protein 27

Cinnamon Cod Mix

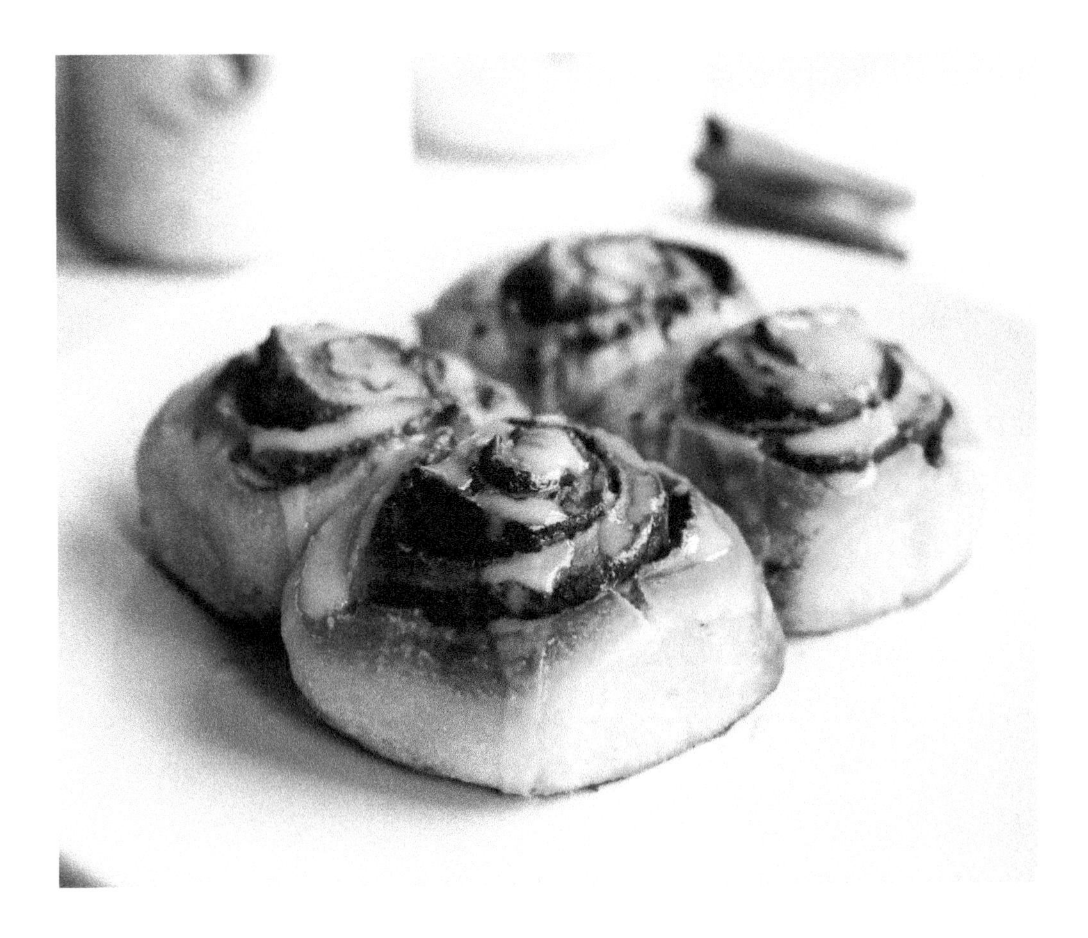

Preparation time: 5 minutes

Cooking time: 12 minutes

Servings: 4

Ingredients:

- 4 cod fillets, boneless and skinless

- 1 tablespoon cinnamon powder
- 1 cup cherry tomatoes, cubed
- Juice of ½ lemon
- ½ cup veggie stock
- A pinch of salt and black pepper
- 1 tablespoon cilantro, chopped

Directions:

In your instant pot, mix the fish with the rest of the ingredients, put the lid on and cook on High for 12 minutes. Release the pressure fast for 5 minutes, divide everything between plates and serve.

Nutrition: calories 162, fat 9.6, fiber 0.3, carbs 3, protein 16.5

Curry Fish

Preparation time: 15 minutes

Cooking time: 4 minutes

Servings: 4

Ingredients:

- 1-pound cod fillet
- 1 teaspoon curry paste
- 2 tablespoons coconut milk
- ½ teaspoon sesame oil
- 1 cup water, for cooking

Directions:

In the shallow bowl whisk together coconut milk and curry paste. Add sesame oil and stir the liquid. After this, chop the cod fillet into the big cubes. Pour the curry mixture over the fish and mix up. Then pour water and insert the steamer rack. Put the fish cubes in the steamer rack and close the lid. Cook the meal on steam mode for 4 minutes. When the time is over, allow the natural pressure release for 5 minutes.

Nutrition: calories 122, fat 4.1, fiber 0.2, carbs 0.8, protein 20.5

Trout and Eggplant Mix

Preparation time: 10 minutes

Cooking time: 15 minutes

Servings: 4

Ingredients:

- 4 trout fillets, boneless
- 2 scallions, chopped
- 2 eggplants, cubed
- ½ cup chicken stock
- 2 tablespoons parsley, chopped
- 3 tablespoons olive oil
- A pinch of salt and black pepper
- 2 tablespoons smoked paprika

Directions:

Set the instant pot on Sauté mode, add the oil, heat it up, add the scallions and the eggplant and cook for 2 minutes, Add the rest of the ingredients except the parsley, put the lid on and cook on High for 13 minutes. Release the pressure naturally for 10 minutes, divide the mix between plates and serve with the parsley sprinkled on top.

Nutrition: calories 291, fat 16.8, fiber 4.5, carbs 6.4, protein 20

Fried Salmon

Preparation time: 10 minutes

Cooking time: 7 minutes

Servings: 4

Ingredients:

- 1 teaspoon Erythritol
- ¼ teaspoon lemongrass
- ¼ teaspoon ground nutmeg
- ½ teaspoon cayenne pepper
- ¼ teaspoon salt
- 1-pound salmon fillet
- 1 tablespoon coconut oil

Directions:

Cut the salmon fillet into 4 fillets. In the shallow bowl combine together spices: lemongrass, ground nutmeg, cayenne pepper, and salt. Rub every salmon fillet with spices. Then toss coconut oil in the instant pot and melt it on sauté mode (approximately 2-3 minutes). Place the salmon fillets in one layer and cook them for 2 minutes from each side. Then sprinkle the salmon fillets with Erythritol and flip on another side. Cook the fish for 1 minute more and transfer in the plate.

Nutrition: calories 181, fat 10.5, fiber 0.1, carbs 1.5, protein 22

Salmon and Tomato Passata

Preparation time: 10 minutes

Cooking time: 15 minutes

Servings: 4

Ingredients:

- 1 tablespoon olive oil
- 4 salmon fillets, boneless, skinless and cubed
- 1 tablespoon rosemary, chopped
- 1 shallot, chopped
- 1 cup tomato passata
- 1 teaspoon chili powder
- 1 tablespoon chives, chopped
- A pinch of salt and black pepper

Directions:

Set the instant pot on Sauté mode, add the oil, heat it up, add the shallot and sauté for 2 minutes. Add the rest of the ingredients, put the lid on and cook on High for 12 minutes. Release the pressure naturally for 10 minutes, divide the mix between plates and serve.

Nutrition: calories 291, fat 16.8, fiber 4.5, carbs 7.4, protein 20

Spicy Mackerel

Preparation time: 15 minutes

Cooking time: 8 minutes

Servings: 4

Ingredients:

- 1-pound fresh mackerel, trimmed
- 1 teaspoon dried oregano
- ½ teaspoon chili powder
- ¼ teaspoon ground black pepper
- ½ teaspoon salt
- ¼ teaspoon chili flakes
- ½ teaspoon dried sage
- 1 teaspoon dried basil

- 1 tablespoon olive oil
- 1 cup water, for cooking

Directions:

In the mixing bowl mix up together dried oregano, chili powder, ground black pepper, salt, chili flakes, dried sage, and dried basil. Then rub the fish with spicy mixture generously. After this, brush it with olive oil and place in the steamer rack, Pour water and insert the steamer rack in the instant pot Close the lid and cook the fish for 8 minutes on Manual mode (high pressure). When the time is over, make a quick pressure release.

Nutrition: calories 330, fat 23.8, fiber 0.3, carbs 0.6, protein 27.2

Salmon and Artichokes

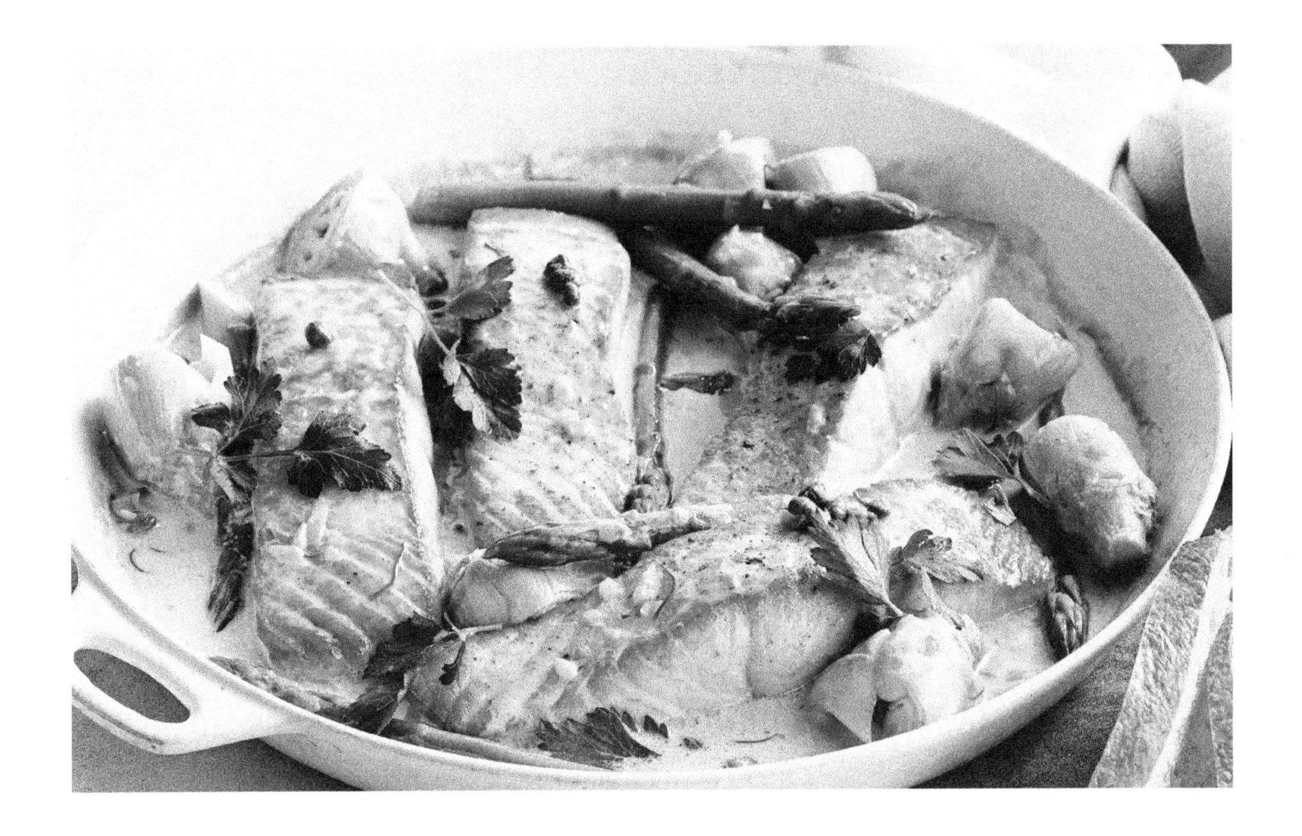

Preparation time: 10 minutes

Cooking time: 15 minutes

Servings: 4

Ingredients:

- 1 pound salmon, skinless, boneless and cubed

- 2 spring onions, chopped
- 12 ounces canned artichokes, roughly chopped
- 1 and ½ cups chicken stock
- A pinch of salt and black pepper
- 1 tablespoon cilantro, chopped

Directions:

In your instant pot, combine all the ingredients, put the lid on and cook on High for 15 minutes. Release the pressure naturally for 10 minutes, divide everything between plates and serve.

Nutrition: calories 193, fat 7.1, fiber 4.1, carbs 6.4, protein 24.5

Salmon in Fragrant Sauce

Preparation time: 10 minutes

Cooking time: 5 minutes

Servings: 2

Ingredients:

- 10 oz salmon fillet
- 1 teaspoon fresh parsley, chopped
- ½ teaspoon lime zest, grated
- 1 teaspoon minced garlic
- 1 jalapeno pepper, diced
- 1 teaspoon Erythritol
- 2 tablespoons avocado oil
- 1 teaspoon ground paprika

- ½ teaspoon ground coriander
- 2 tablespoons lemon juice
- 1 cup water, for cooking

Directions:

Cut the salmon fillet into 2 servings. Pour water and insert the steamer rack in the instant pot. Place the salmon fillets on the rack and close the lid. Steam the fish for 5 minutes on Steam mode. When the time is over make a quick pressure release and transfer the fish on the plates. While the fish is cooking, make the fragrant sauce: in the bowl combine together parsley, lime zest, minced garlic, diced jalapeno pepper, Erythritol, avocado oil, paprika, ground coriander, and lemon juice. Pour the sauce over the cooked salmon.

Nutrition: calories 218, fat 10.8, fiber 1.4, carbs 5.2, protein 28.2

Trout and Spinach Mix

Preparation time: 5 minutes

Cooking time: 15 minutes

Servings: 4

Ingredients:

- 6 trout fillets, boneless
- 2 tablespoons avocado oil
- 2 scallions, minced
- 2 garlic cloves, minced
- 2 tablespoons cilantro, chopped
- 1 cup baby spinach
- A pinch of salt and black pepper
- 2 tablespoons balsamic vinegar

Directions:

Set the instant pot on Sauté mode, add the oil, heat it up, add the scallions and the garlic and sauté for 2 minutes. Add the rest of the ingredients, put the lid on and cook on High for 12 minutes. Release the pressure fast for 5 minutes, divide the mix between plates and serve.

Nutrition: calories 194, fat 8.8, fiber 0.7, carbs 1.8, protein 25.4

Shrimp Salad with Avocado

Preparation time: 10 minutes

Cooking time: 7 minutes

Servings: 4

Ingredients:

- ½ avocado, chopped
- 7 oz shrimps, peeled
- 1 cup lettuce, chopped
- 2 bacon slices, chopped
- 2 tablespoons heavy cream
- 1 teaspoon peanuts, chopped
- ½ teaspoon ground black pepper
- ¼ teaspoon Pink salt

- 1 cup water, for cooking

Directions:

Pour water and insert the steamer rack in the instant pot. Place the shrimps in the rack and close the lid. Cook them on manual mode (high pressure) for 1 minute. Then make quick pressure release and transfer the shrimps in the salad bowl. Remove the steamer rack and clean the instant pot bowl. Place the bacon in the instant pot and cook it on sauté mode for 6 minutes. Stir it every minute to avoid burning. Then transfer the cooked bacon to the shrimps. Add chopped bacon, lettuce, and peanuts. Then in the shallow bowl mix up together heavy cream, peanuts, ground black pepper, and Pink salt. Pour the liquid over the salad and shake it gently.

Nutrition: calories 194, fat 12.9, fiber 1.9, carbs 4, protein 15.7

Sea Bass and Sauce

Preparation time: 10 minutes

Cooking time: 15 minutes

Servings: 4

Ingredients:

- 4 sea bass fillets, boneless and skinless
- 2 tablespoons lime juice
- 2 garlic cloves, minced
- 1 shallot, chopped
- 1 cup chicken stock
- 1 cup tomato passata
- A pinch of salt and black pepper

Directions:

In your instant pot, combine the fish with the rest of the ingredients, put the lid on and cook on High for 15 minutes. Release the pressure naturally for 10 minutes, divide the mix between plates and serve.

Nutrition: calories 154, fat 2.9, fiber 1.3, carbs 2.5, protein 25

Seafood Omelet

Preparation time: 15 minutes

Cooking time: 10 minutes

Servings:4

Ingredients:

- 4 eggs, beaten
- 2 tablespoons cream cheese
- ½ teaspoon chili flakes
- 1 oz Parmesan, grated
- 5 oz crab meat, canned, chopped
- ½ teaspoon butter, melted
- 1 teaspoon chives, chopped
- 1 cup water, for cooking

Directions:

In the mixing bowl combine together eggs, cream cheese, chili flakes, and chives. Brush the instant pot baking pan with butter and pour the egg mixture inside. Top the egg mixture with chopped crab meat and grated Parmesan. Whisk the mixture gently with the help of the fork. Pour water and insert the steamer rack in the instant pot. Place the instant pot baking pan in the rack and close the lid. Cook the omelet on steam mode for 10 minutes. When the time is over, allow the natural pressure release for 5 minutes.

Nutrition: calories 139, fat 8.7, fiber 0, carbs 1.4, protein 12.7

Sea Bass and Pesto

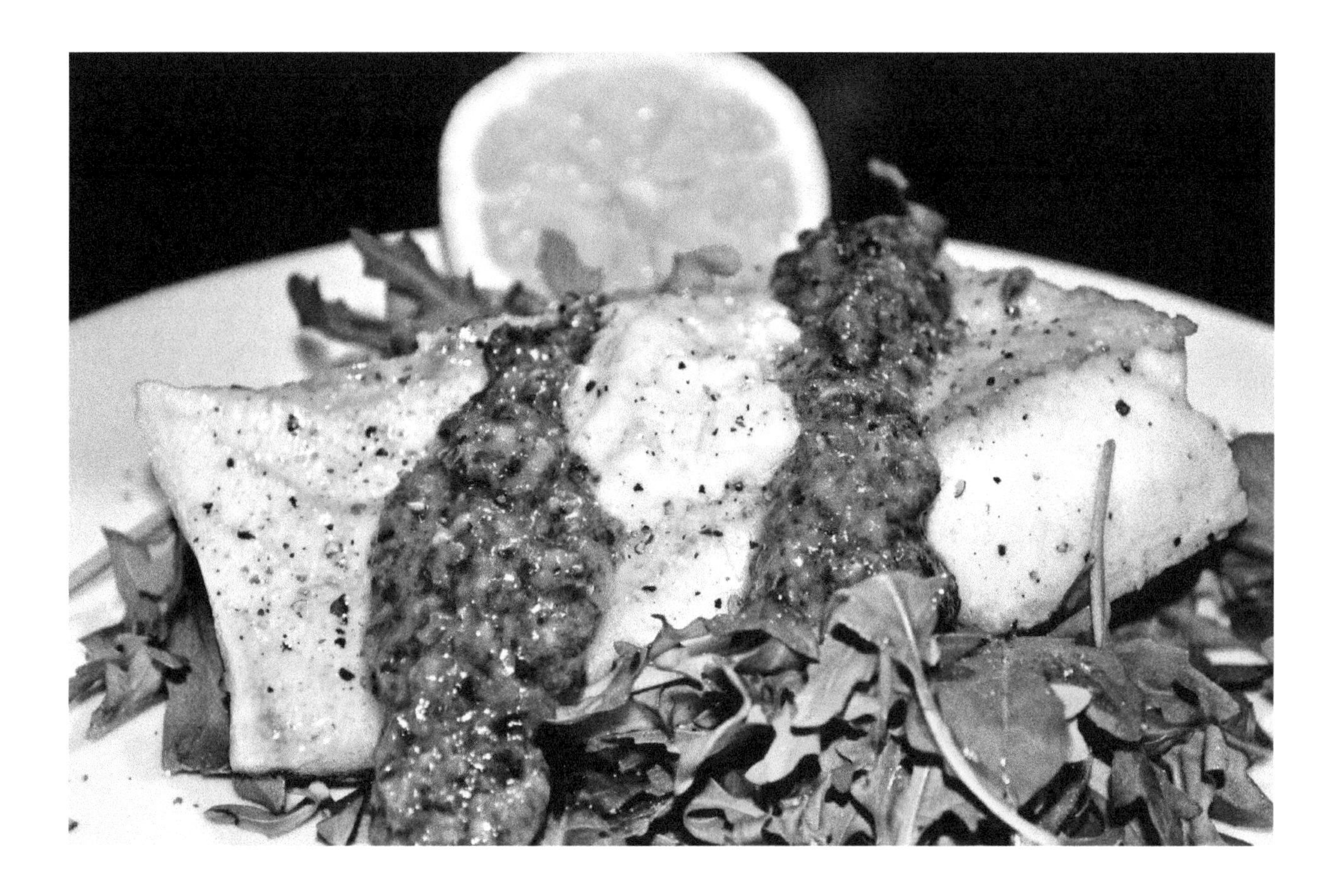

Preparation time: 5 minutes

Cooking time: 12 minutes

Servings: 4

Ingredients:

- 4 sea bass fillets, skinless, boneless
- 2 tablespoons olive oil
- 2 tablespoons garlic, chopped
- 1 cup basil, chopped
- 2 tablespoons pine nuts
- A pinch of salt and black pepper
- 1 cup tomato passata
- 1 tablespoon parsley, chopped

Directions:

In your blender, combine the oil with the garlic, basil, pine nuts, slat and pepper and pulse well. In your instant pot, combine the sea bass with the pesto, salt, pepper, tomato passata and the parsley, put the lid on and cook on High for 12 minutes. Release the pressure fast for 5 minutes, divide the mix between plates and serve.

Nutrition: calories 237, fat 12.7, fiber 1.3, carbs 5.5, protein 25.8

Shrimp Tacos

Preparation time: 10 minutes

Cooking time: 1 minute

Servings:5

Ingredients:

- 5 low carb tortillas
- ½ cup white cabbage, shredded
- 2 oz Cotija cheese, crumbled
- 1 tablespoon lemon juice
- ½ teaspoon ground cumin
- ½ teaspoon cayenne pepper
- ¼ teaspoon garlic powder
- ¼ teaspoon onion powder

- ½ teaspoon chili powder
- 1 tablespoon green onions, chopped
- 1 tablespoon fresh cilantro, chopped
- 2 tablespoons avocado oil
- 3 tablespoons heavy cream
- 1-pound shrimps, peeled
- 1 cup water, for cooking

Directions:

Pour water and insert the steamer rack in the instant pot. In the mixing bowl combine together lemon juice, ground cumin, cayenne pepper, garlic powder, onion powder, and chili powder. Coat the shrimps in the mixture and transfer in the steamer rack. Close the lid and cook them for 1 minute on Manual mode (high pressure). Make a quick pressure release and open the lid. Make the taco sauce: mix up together heavy cream, avocado oil, cilantro, and green onions. Then mix up together shredded white cabbage and sauce. Place the cooked shrimps on the tortillas. Add shredded cabbage mixture and Cotija cheese. Fold the tortillas into the tacos.

Nutrition: calories 272, fat 10.9, fiber 7.7, carbs 15, protein 27

Tuna and Mustard Greens

Preparation time: 10 minutes

Cooking time: 10 minutes

Servings: 4

Ingredients:

- 2 cups mustard greens
- 1 tablespoon olive oil
- 1 cup tomato passata
- 1 shallot, chopped
- 1 tablespoon basil, chopped
- A pinch of salt and black pepper
- 14 ounces tuna fillets, boneless, skinless and cubed

Directions:

Set your instant pot on Sauté mode, add the oil, heat it up, add the shallot and sauté for 2 minutes. Add rest of the ingredients, put the lid on and cook on High for 8 minutes. Release the pressure naturally for 10 minutes, divide the mix between plates and serve.

Nutrition: calories 124, fat 3.7, fiber 1.9, carbs 2.6, protein 1.6

Shrimp Cocktail

Preparation time: 10 minutes

Cooking time: 1 minute

Servings: 6

Ingredients:

- 16 oz shrimps, peeled
- 1 cup low carb ketchup
- ½ tablespoon lemon juice
- 1 teaspoon horseradish, grated
- ¼ teaspoon white pepper
- ½ teaspoon salt
- 1 cup water, for cooking

Directions:

Pour water and insert the steamer rack in the instant pot. Sprinkle the shrimps with salt and place in the steamer rack. Cook the seafood for 0 minutes on manual mode (high pressure). Make a quick pressure release and transfer the shrimps in the serving plate. Then make shrimp cocktail sauce: in the sauce bowl, mix up together low carb ketchup, lemon juice, horseradish, and white pepper. Dip the shrimps in the sauce.

Nutrition: calories 99, fat 1.3, fiber 0.1, carbs 1.3, protein 17.3

Salmon and Salsa

Preparation time: 10 minutes

Cooking time: 8 minutes

Servings: 4

Ingredients:

- 4 salmon fillets, boneless
- ½ cup veggie stock
- 1 cup black olives, pitted
- 1 cup tomatoes, cubed
- 1 tablespoon basil, chopped
- 1 tablespoon olive oil
- 1 tablespoon balsamic vinegar
- A pinch of salt and black pepper

- 1 tablespoon chives, chopped

Directions:

In your instant pot, combine the fish with the stock, salt and pepper, put the lid on and cook on High for 8 minutes. Release the pressure naturally for 10 minutes and divide the salmon between plates. In a bowl, mix the olives with the rest of the ingredients, toss, add next to the salmon and serve.

Nutrition: calories 313, fat 18.2, fiber 1.7, carbs 4, protein 35.4

Mussels Casserole

Preparation time: 10 minutes

Cooking time: 13 minutes

Servings: 4

Ingredients:

- 9 oz mussels, canned
- 1 cup cauliflower, chopped
- ½ cup Cheddar cheese, shredded
- ½ cup heavy cream
- 1 teaspoon Italian seasonings
- 1 teaspoon olive oil
- 1 teaspoon salt
- 1 tablespoon fresh dill, chopped

- 1 cup water, for cooking

Directions:

Pour water and insert the trivet in the instant pot. Place the cauliflower on the trivet and cook it on manual mode (high pressure) for 3 minutes. Then make a quick pressure release. Transfer the cauliflower in the instant pot casserole mold. Add canned mussels, cheese, heavy cream, Italian seasonings, olive oil, salt, and dill. Mix up the casserole and cover it with foil. Place the casserole mold on the trivet and close the lid. Cook the casserole for 10 minutes on manual mode (high pressure). When the time is over, make a quick pressure release. Mix up the casserole with the help of the spoon before serving.

Nutrition: calories 185, fat 13.2, fiber 0.7, carbs 4.9, protein 12.1

Saffron Chili Cod

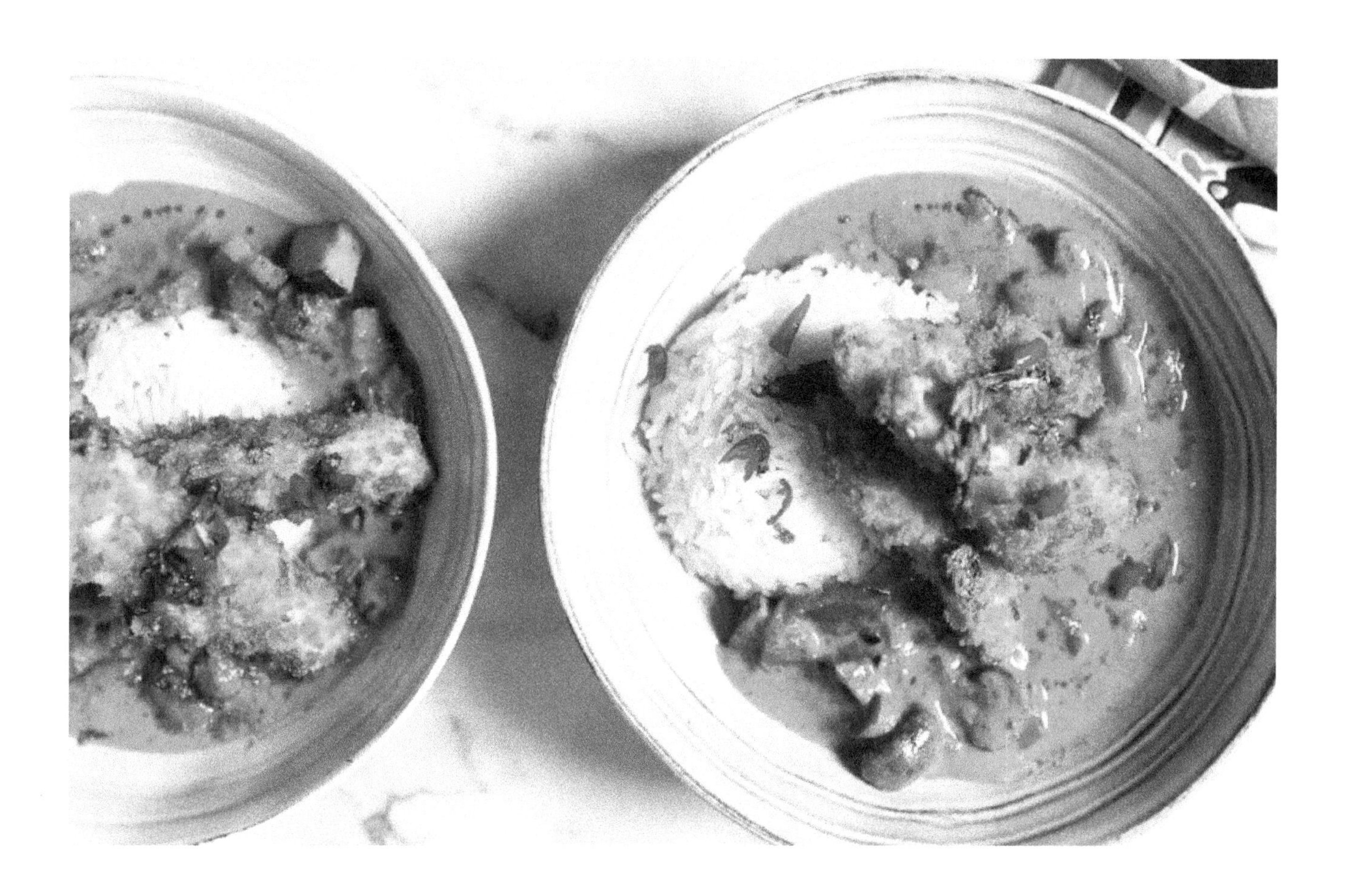

Preparation time: 5 minutes

Cooking time: 12 minutes

Servings: 4

Ingredients:

- 4 cod fillets, boneless and skinless
- 3 garlic cloves, minced
- 1 teaspoon turmeric powder
- 1 tablespoon chili paste
- 1 cup tomato passata

Directions:

In your instant pot, combine the cod with the rest of the ingredients, put the lid on and cook on High for 12 minutes. Release the pressure fast for 5 minutes, divide everything between plates and serve.

Nutrition: calories 244, fat 12, fiber 1.6, carbs 4.5, protein 14.6

Skagenrora

Preparation time: 10 minutes

Cooking time: 1 minute

Servings:4

Ingredients:

- 11 oz shrimps, peeled
- ½ cup of coconut milk
- 1 tablespoon ricotta cheese
- 2 tablespoons fresh parsley, chopped
- 1 teaspoon lime juice
- ¼ teaspoon chili powder
- ¼ teaspoon ground black pepper
- 1 red onion, chopped

- 1 cup water, for cooking

Directions:

Pour water and insert the steamer rack in the instant pot. Put the shrimps in the rack and close the lid. Cook them on manual mode (high pressure) for 1 minute. When the time is over, make a quick pressure release and transfer the shrimps in the salad bowl. In the separated bowl mix up together coconut milk, ricotta cheese, fresh parsley, lime juice, chili powder, and ground black pepper. The sauce is cooked. Combine together shrimps with chopped red onion. Add sauce and mix it up.

Nutrition: calories 180, fat 8.9, fiber 1.4, carbs 6, protein 19.3

Salmon and Endives

Preparation time: 10 minutes

Cooking time: 15 minutes

Servings: 4

Ingredients:

- 4 salmon fillets, boneless
- 1 cup tomato passata
- 1 shallot, sliced
- 2 endives, trimmed and halved
- 1 tablespoon balsamic vinegar
- A pinch of salt and black pepper
- 1 tablespoon parsley, chopped

Directions:

In your instant pot, combine the salmon with the rest of the ingredients, put the lid on and cook on High for 15 minutes. Release the pressure naturally for 10 minutes, divide the mix between plates and serve.

Nutrition: calories 251, fat 11.1, fiber 1, carbs 3.4, protein 35.4

Butter Scallops

Preparation time: 10 minutes

Cooking time: 7 minutes

Servings: 4

Ingredients:

- 1-pound scallops
- 3 tablespoons butter
- ½ teaspoon dried rosemary
- ¼ teaspoon salt

Directions:

Put butter in the instant pot. Set sauté mode and melt butter (it will take approximately 3 minutes. Add dried rosemary and salt. Stir the butter. Then place the scallops in the hot butter in one layer. Cook them on sauté mode for 2 minutes. Then flip the scallops on another side and cook for 2 minutes more. Serve the scallops with hot butter.

Nutrition: calories 177, fat 9.5, fiber 0.1, carbs 2.8, protein 19.1

Chili Tuna

Preparation time: 5 minutes

Cooking time: 15 minutes

Servings: 4

Ingredients:

- 1 pound tuna, skinless, boneless and cubed
- Juice of 1 lemon
- 1 tablespoon chili powder
- 1 cup tomato passata
- A pinch of salt and black pepper
- 1 shallot, chopped
- 1 tablespoon chives, chopped
- 1 tablespoon cilantro, chopped

Directions:

In your instant pot, combine the tuna with the lemon juice and the rest of the ingredients, put the lid on and cook on High for 15 minutes. Release the pressure fast for 5 minutes, divide the chili into bowls and serve.

Nutrition: calories 232, fat 9.6, fiber 1.6, carbs 4.4, protein 31.2

Cajun Crab Casserole

Preparation time: 10 minutes

Cooking time: 15 minutes

Servings: 6

Ingredients:

- ½ cup celery stalks, chopped
- ½ white onion, diced
- 3 eggs, beaten
- 1 tablespoon dried parsley
- 10 oz crab meat, chopped, canned
- 1 teaspoon Cajun seasonings
- ½ cup white Cheddar cheese, shredded
- ½ teaspoon salt

- ½ teaspoon ground black pepper
- ½ teaspoon cayenne pepper
- ½ cup heavy cream
- 1 teaspoon sesame oil

Directions:

Heat up the instant pot on sauté mode for 3 minutes and add sesame oil. Add diced onion and cook it for 2 minutes. Stir it well. Switch off the instant pot. Add celery stalk in the onion and mix up. Then add beaten eggs, dried parsley, crab meat, Cajun seasonings, cheese, salt, ground black pepper, cayenne pepper, and heavy cream. Stir the casserole carefully with the help of a spatula and close the lid. Cook the meal on stew mode for 10 minutes.

Nutrition: calories 159, fat 9.7, fiber 0.4, carbs 2.8, protein 11.5

Mackerel and Shrimp Mix

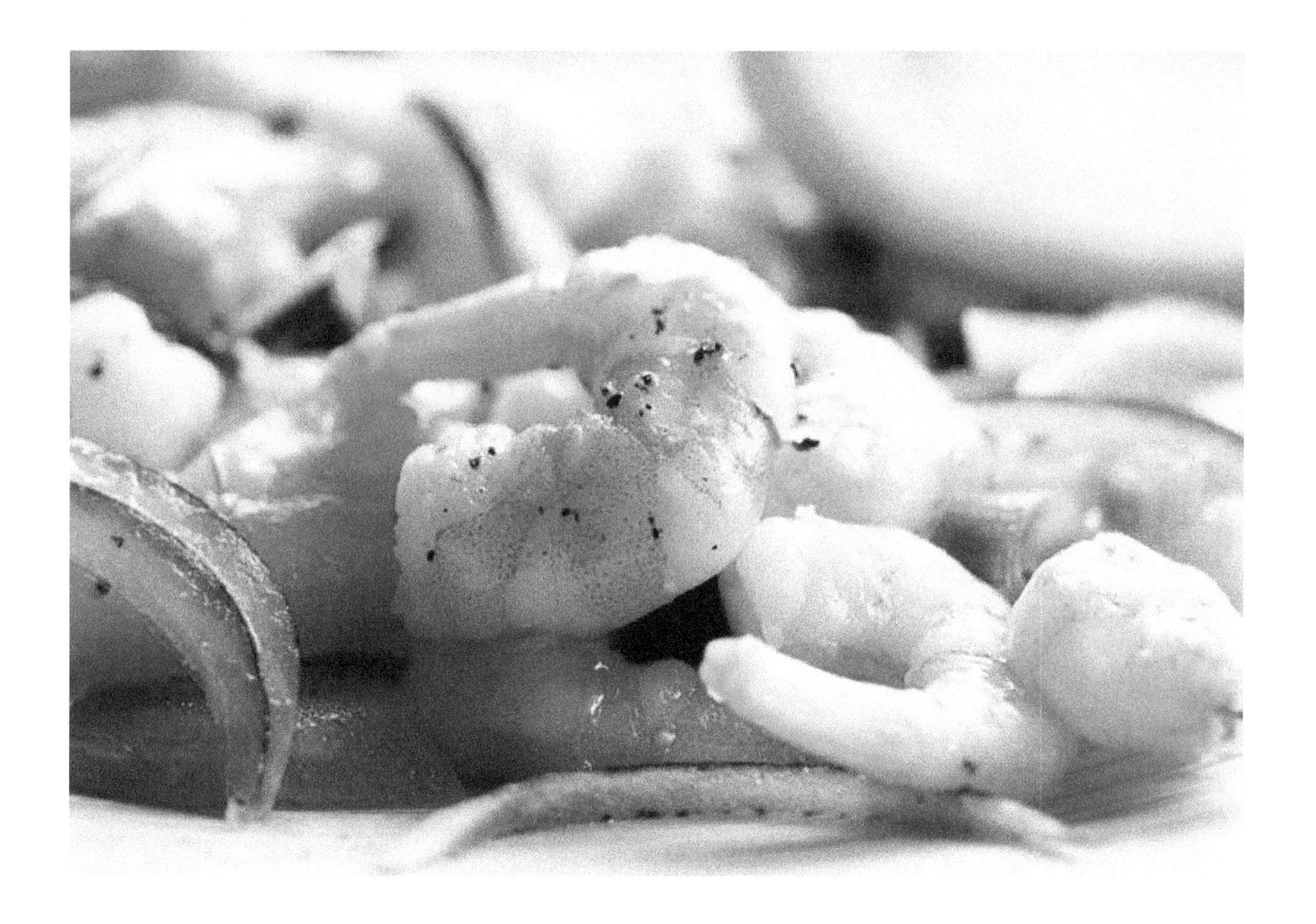

Preparation time: 5 minutes

Cooking time: 12 minutes

Servings: 6

Ingredients:

- 1 pound shrimp, peeled and deveined
- 1 pound mackerel, skinless, boneless and cubed
- 1 cup radishes, cubed
- ½ cup chicken stock
- 2 garlic cloves, minced
- 1 tablespoon olive oil
- 1 cup tomato passata

Directions:

Set instant pot on Sauté mode, add the oil, heat it up, add the radishes and the garlic and sauté for 2 minutes. Add the rest of the ingredients, put the lid on and cook on High for 10 minutes. Release the pressure fast for 5 minutes, divide the mix into bowls and serve.

Nutrition: calories 332, fat 17.4, fiber 0.9, carbs 4.4, protein 36.4

Crab Melt with Zucchini

Preparation time: 15 minutes

Cooking time: 8 minutes

Servings: 4

Ingredients:

- 1 large zucchini
- 1 teaspoon avocado oil
- ½ cup Monterey Jack cheese, shredded
- 1 green bell pepper, finely chopped
- 9 oz crab meat, chopped
- 2 tablespoons ricotta cheese
- 1 cup water, for cooking

Directions:

Trim the ends of zucchini and slice it lengthwise into 4 slices. Then pour water in the instant pot and insert the trivet. Place the zucchini slices in the baking mold. Brush them with avocado oil gently. After this, in the mixing bowl combine together Monterey Jack cheese, bell pepper, crab meat, and ricotta cheese. Spread the mixture over the zucchini and transfer it on the trivet. Close the instant pot lid and cook the meal on manual mode (high pressure) for 8 minutes. When the time is over, make a quick pressure release.

Nutrition: calories 144, fat 6.4, fiber 1.3, carbs 6.7, protein 13.6

Mackerel and Basil Sauce

Preparation time: 10 minutes

Cooking time: 15 minutes

Servings: 4

Ingredients:

- 1 cup veggie stock
- 2 chili peppers, chopped
- 2 tablespoons olive oil
- 1 pound mackerel, skinless, boneless and cubed
- 2 teaspoons red pepper flakes
- A pinch of salt and black pepper
- ½ cup basil, chopped

Directions:

Set your instant pot on Sauté mode, add the oil, heat it up, add the chili peppers and the pepper flakes and cook for 2 minutes. Add the rest of the ingredients, put the lid on and cook on High for 12 minutes. Release the pressure naturally for 10 minutes, divide everything between plates and serve.

Nutrition: calories 362, fat 14.7, fiber 0.4, carbs 0.8, protein 27.5

Baked Snapper

Preparation time: 10 minutes

Cooking time: 10 minutes

Servings: 4

Ingredients:

- 1-pound snapper, trimmed, cleaned
- 1 tablespoon lemongrass
- 1 tablespoon sage
- 1 teaspoon avocado oil
- 1 teaspoon salt
- 1 teaspoon red pepper
- 1 cup water, for cooking

Directions:

Pour water and insert trivet in the instant pot. Rub the fish with salt and red pepper. Then fill it with sage and lemongrass. Brush the fish with avocado oil and transfer on the trivet. Close the lid and cook the snapper for 10 minutes on manual mode (high pressure). When the time is over, make a quick pressure release and open the lid. Remove the sage and lemongrass from the fish.

Nutrition: calories 151, fat 2.2, fiber 0.7, carbs 2.9, protein 27.9

Oregano Tuna

Preparation time: 10 minutes

Cooking time: 12 minutes

Servings: 4

Ingredients:

- 1 pound tuna, skinless, boneless and cubed
- 1 cup black olives, pitted and sliced
- 2 tablespoon avocado oil
- 1 shallot, chopped
- 14 ounces tomatoes, chopped
- 2 tablespoons oregano, chopped

Directions:

Set your instant pot on Sauté mode, add the oil, heat it up, add the shallot and sauté for 2 minutes. Add the tuna and the rest of the ingredients, put the lid on and cook on High for 10 minutes. Release the pressure naturally for 10 minutes, divide the mix between plates and serve.

Nutrition: calories 284, fat 14.1, fiber 3.5, carbs 6.7, protein 31.4

Salmon Salad

Preparation time: 10 minutes

Cooking time: 8 minutes

Servings: 2

Ingredients:

- ½ cup curly kale, chopped
- 7 oz salmon fillet, chopped
- 1 teaspoon onion flakes
- ½ teaspoon salt
- 1 teaspoon coconut oil
- 1 teaspoon olive oil
- ½ teaspoon chili flakes
- ¼ cup cherry tomatoes, halved

Directions:

Place coconut oil in the instant pot and heat it up on sauté mode. When the coconut oil is melted, add salmon fillet. Sprinkle the fish with salt and chili flakes. Cook it for 2 minutes from each side on sauté mode. Then transfer the cooked salmon in the salad bowl. Add curly kale, onion flakes, salt, olive oil, and halved cherry tomatoes. Shake the salad.

Nutrition: calories 202, fat 11.2, fiber 2.2, carbs 6, protein 21.7

Conclusion

The instant pot is such a cutting-edge and advanced cooking tool. It has gained a lot of fans throughout the world. The instant pot permits you to cook delicious dishes for all your household in a matter of minutes and with minimal initiative. The most effective thing about the instant pot is that you do not need to be a professional cook to make tasty culinary feasts. You just need the best components and also the right instructions. That's exactly how you'll obtain the most effective instant pot dishes.

This wonderful cooking guide you have actually simply uncovered is more than a basic instant pot food preparation journal. It is a Ketogenic split second pot recipes collection you will discover really beneficial.

The Ketogenic diet plan will provide you the energy increase you require, it will make you lose the additional weight and also it will certainly improve your general health in a matter of days. This collection has the most effective Ketogenic immediate pot meals you can prepare in the convenience of your own residence. All these recipes are so flavorful as well as textured and they all taste extraordinary.

So, if you are adhering to a Ketogenic diet plan and also you own an instantaneous pot, get your own duplicate of this cookbook and also begin your Ketogenic culinary adventure. Cook the most effective Ketogenic split second pot dishes and enjoy them all!